THIN THIGHS
in **30** *Days*

www.**rbooks**.co.uk

THIN THIGHS
in **30** *Days*

WENDY STEHLING

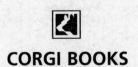

CORGI BOOKS

TRANSWORLD PUBLISHERS
61–63 Uxbridge Road, London W5 5SA
A Random House Group Company
www.rbooks.co.uk

THIN THIGHS IN 30 DAYS
A CORGI BOOK: 9780552164054

Previously published in 1982 by Bantam Books, Inc.
This revised and updated edition first published by the Penguin Group (USA) Inc.
Corgi edition published 2011

A CIP catalogue record for this book
is available from the British Library.

Addresses for Random House Group Ltd companies outside the UK
can be found at: www.randomhouse.co.uk
The Random House Group Ltd Reg. No. 954009

The Random House Group Limited supports The Forest Stewardship Council
(FSC), the leading international forest certification organisation. All our titles that
are printed on Greenpeace approved FSC certified paper carry the FSC logo. Our
paper procurement policy can be found at
www.rbooks.co.uk/environment

Typeset in 11/16pt Giovanni by Falcon Oast Graphic Art Ltd.
Printed in the UK by CPI Cox & Wyman, Reading, RG1 8EX.

2 4 6 8 10 9 7 5 3 1

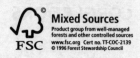

To my mother—with her amazing grace.
To my father, who always urged me to write.
To 'lil bro, love you.

Contents

Dear Beautiful New Friend:

Have you ever had this experience?

I tried on a favorite pair of pants I had not put on in a year. Groan. I was pretty sure that if I tried to sit down—the seams would pop!

Somehow over the course of the year, some inches had crept onto my thighs. How had this happened? Well, I couldn't blame it on "winter weight"—it was May! How about my age? (I'm fifty-nine.) I knew plenty of women my age or well over it who had thin and supple thighs, so there was no excuse for me! Who could say why these inches had appeared on my thighs? The good news is that I knew the perfect program to take them off; heck, I'd written a whole book on the subject—a book that sold

2.5 million copies when it was originally published back in 1982.

Back when I first designed the Thin Thighs in 30 Days program, I had had a rough encounter with a department store three-way mirror and a bright pink bathing suit—similar to my encounter with that favorite pair of pants—and I was looking for some serious help! I was in the advertising business at the time, which brought me into constant contact with models and celebrities who were quite serious about keeping their thighs sleek and beautiful. I embarked on a project to learn about these beautiful women's methods for keeping their thighs slender and lovely. I spoke to their doctors and beauty advisers, and then tested the program on myself and other women.

The original Thin Thighs program is (and had to be) tough, because thighs are tough to reduce. But the results were indisputable: In just one month, women who read the book and followed the program had thinner, firmer thighs. I knew it was a program that really worked, but it had been twenty-seven years since I'd designed it, and, to be honest, while I'd kept it up pretty consistently over the years, the last year had been a tough one and I'd managed to pile a few unwanted pounds onto my thighs. I decided to take a look at my old program and study up on the latest diet and fitness research, and guess what? It was still solid. Sometimes the best advice really is the simplest, *and* Thin Thighs in 30 Days *is certainly a case in point. With just a few updates here and there . . . voilà! You are now holding in your hands a new and improved version of my classic thigh-thinning program, Thin Thighs in 30 Days!*

This revised and updated version of Thin Thighs in 30 Days *incorporates all of the latest information about safe and effective exercise and weight loss into the original, tried-and-true Thin Thighs program. The original program consisted of just three parts: The Work-Off, The Walk-Off, and The Weight-Off, and this revised program is still built around this clear and effective three-pronged approach. I've just added in a few new killer exercises that, believe me, I know work! Also new to the program: three separate programs that meet you right where you are in terms of fitness (beginner, intermediate, and advanced) and an interval training component so you can get even more bang for your exercise buck.*

With this book I invite you to do something that I promise will get your thighs lean and sexy—and fast. So without further ado, let's get started!

First, *I want you to measure your thighs at the "biggest" point. Before I started the program, mine measured 25 ½ inches. Now weigh yourself—I weighed in at 142 ½ pounds (I am five feet, seven inches tall).*

Second, *focus on your goal! After I followed my 30-day program, my thighs thinned to 23 ¼ inches, and* my weight dropped to 131 pounds. And I was never hungry! In fact, by focusing on thigh-thinning exercise and good eating, I felt better than ever. Plus, the long-term benefits to my health are enormous.

And the pants fit.

So think big (or, in this case, small!), and get ready to start right away. This fun, focused, 30-day program will guarantee that in just one month you will have the most beautiful thin thighs ever!

Love,
Wendy

Spring 2010

P.S. Before you start this diet and exercise program, be sure to get the approval of your doctor or health-care practitioner.

Introduction

|||||||||||||||||||||||||||||||||||||||||||||||||||||||||||||||||||||||

This is your lucky day! No matter what your bone structure or body shape, you can have firmer, thinner thighs. Fighting back against gravity, you will eliminate bulges and sags and ultimately look sleeker in pants, shorts, dresses, and bathing suits.

Most important, there are many health benefits to the Thin Thighs in 30 Days program. Exercise and healthy eating give you heart health and stronger bones, reduce the risk of diabetes and varicose veins, may boost your immune system, and can even improve your brainpower! Plus, you will have more energy to do your daily errands—

or maybe dance all night (which is also great for your thighs!).

Your results can be judged by your appearance and how you feel—as well as with a tape measure (a cut-out tape measure is included at the back of the book, or you can find one at your local drugstore). Twice a week, measure the same thigh in the same place (ideally just below your bum at the thigh's largest area). Remember, even an inch or two lost will make a big difference in your appearance.

Assuming you may need to eat less to get to your target weight (and most of us will), weigh yourself before you begin the program. Then weigh yourself at least once a week, first thing in the morning. You will be burning calories and the pounds will melt—the Weight-Off really works!

Have fun focusing on your body, not just for 30 days but for a lifetime! You will find that once you are in the habit of being focused on feel-good activities, not to mention the love affair you'll be having with your sleek and sexy thighs, you will want to continue to keep yourself healthy and beautiful!

Get Ready to Start on Saturday

When it comes to making your thighs thinner, there's no time to start like the present. I encourage you to begin your program this next Saturday. Because I know how hard it sometimes can be to embark upon a new project, let me try to make it less intimidating for you by laying out the very first four steps you should take:

FIRST: FOCUS on your goal: thinner thighs.

SECOND: COMMIT to devoting at least 1 hour each day to your thighs. Agree you will do the Work-Off and Walk-Off faithfully six days each week (sorry, ladies, the Weight-Off must be followed every day, seven days a week, for the entire 30 days!). You wouldn't skip brushing your teeth for a day, so why not place the same importance on your thighs! Monday should be your rest from exercise day. You can alter the week if you'd like, but keep the same pattern throughout the 30 days.

THIRD: If you determine that you'll need to lose weight in order to really slim your thighs down to the desired size, AGREE to eat fewer calories. Think about everything you put into your mouth!

FOUR: This book includes three very effective programs that work *synergistically* to give you thin thighs: the Work-Off, the Walk-Off, and the Weight-Off. Commit to doing all three diligently if you are serious about wanting thin thighs!

Make no excuses and allow no interruptions! If you travel, find a way to do this program while you are away. Remember to take your running shoes and pack an appropriate outfit. Pick a time for your Walk-Off and Work-Off and be as regular with that time as possible. Maybe you like to get up very early and thin your thighs in the fresh air of dawn, or you may want to unwind and recharge with exercise at the end of the day. Or use your lunch hour for a great escape!

Most important, have fun!

What You Need to Get Started

You will need these simple items of equipment to get started:

- Your Thin Thighs in 30 Days diary and a pen or pencil
- Measuring tape (see back of book, or purchase one in a store)

- Scale (optional)
- The best pair of running/walking shoes you can afford. Go to a running store if you can, and be sure you buy shoes that aren't too tight (I wear men's shoes so that I have ample room for my feet). There should be at least a thumbnail from your big toe to the end of the sole.
- Jog bra (especially if you will be incorporating jogging into your Walk-Off program)
- Comfortable clothes for the Walk-Off, and any type of clothing or nothing for the Work-Off

HOW TO USE THIS BOOK

The new and improved *Thin Thighs in 30 Days* allows you to tailor your program to where you are right now in terms of your fitness level. Use the following guidelines to determine if you should undergo a beginner, intermediate, or advanced Thin Thighs program.

Assess Your Current Level of Fitness

Which one are you?

> **BEGINNER:** You currently do not follow a regular cardiovascular program (walking, skating, running, tennis, etc.). By regular, I mean 3 times a week for at least 30 minutes.
>
> **INTERMEDIATE:** You walk/run or participate in another cardiovascular workout at least 3 times a week for 30 minutes or more. You can walk a 13-minute mile. You can walk at least 2 to 3 miles at a brisk pace comfortably.
>
> **ADVANCED:** You walk/run or participate in another cardiovascular workout at least 5 times a week for 30 minutes or more. You can walk a 12-minute mile. You can walk/run for 5 or more miles at a brisk pace comfortably.

After participating in my program for 30 days, you will condition yourself to a new level!

FINDING YOUR SPECIFIC GOALS
AND CHARTING YOUR PROGRESS

Following a guide and tracking your progress toward thinner thighs will help keep you focused. Ideally, you will *get into the habit* of keeping your thighs in shape, maintaining an ideal weight, and working to keep your heart and body healthy. In the meantime, the Daily Diaries included in the back of this book provide you with a place to chart your specific 30-day goals and note your individual progress. Think of them as your day-by-day progress reports.

Within each of the Diaries (Beginner, Intermediate, and Advanced), you will find specific goals and places to check off that you have accomplished them. For the Work-Off portion of the diaries, you will notice that everyone, at all fitness levels, has the same starting number of repetitions and goal. This is because these leg exercises are very focused, and they can make you sore. So ease into them. You'll see, they work. In the Walk-Off portions of the diaries, you will note specific walking and/or jogging goals in terms of duration and intensity based on your own particular fitness level for each week of the program.

If you feel like pushing beyond what is directed in the Diaries, do so only if you feel good. This said, the recommendations made are on the safe side—if you feel like pushing yourself, go ahead!

Here are a few tips for using the diaries:

- Start on a Saturday.
- Every day enter what you've done. If you skipped a day, write nothing. And remember that you need to make up that day. NO EXCUSES, please! You should only skip a day if you are too ill to participate or dangerous weather conditions exist.
- Be proud as you fill up the diary.
- Monday is your day off from exercise —but remember to continue watching what you eat carefully.
- Have fun! Each day you will be more beautiful and healthier. Not to mention the fact that all those around you will soon be envious of your thin thighs!

THIN THIGHS IN 30 DAYS EXPRESS

With this new and improved version of *Thin Thighs in 30 Days*, it is now possible to speed up your results—lose inches faster, have firmer, sleeker thighs sooner. This new supplemental program is in the back of the book (see page 105). DOUBLE UP on your daily Thin Thighs in 30 Days program. You can choose how many days a week to do this. Bottom line— when you exercise more often, you become fit faster!

THE BASIC SCHEDULE

Regardless of your fitness level, this program is designed to make you work hard all week but also to rest. Varying the intensity of your exercise program is essential so that you can keep your stamina going and also so that you can allow muscle to strengthen. Here is an overview of the 30-day schedule:

SATURDAY: Easy effort
SUNDAY: Longest effort to increase endurance
MONDAY: Day off
TUESDAY: Intervals for cardiovascular workout
    and to improve technique
WEDNESDAY: Moderate effort
THURSDAY: Moderate effort
FRIDAY: Intense effort (hills and/or intervals)
    to improve strength

Let's get started!

The Work-Off

||||||||||||||||||||||||||||||||||||||||||||||||||||||||||||||||||||||||||

don't have naturally thin thighs—I have a long, thin neck and long dangly arms, but my legs have been politely referred to as "athletic". I am not alone: Most women have a wide pelvic area designed for bearing children, and chances are excess fat shows up on your hips and thighs. The good news is that with focused diet and exercise, we can eliminate some of that fat and firm things up quite a bit!

Look at yourself in the mirror in your underwear. What do you see? A few jiggly bits, or even those dreaded saddle-bags? What about pudgy lumps on your inner thighs? Is your bum sort of drooping? I don't mean to sound depressing; I am just commiserating. But remember, we can do something about it!

Periods of extended inactivity cause muscles to lose their tone. Since most of us sit for many hours each day (can't you just feel your thighs spreading on the chair?), the Work-Off is an important part of getting your thighs to be strong, lean, and trim.

HOW TO DO THE WORK-OFF EXERCISES

First, I'm going to ask you to do something that might sound unusual in relationship to exercise: feel happy about these floor exercises. They actually are not boring or tedious. Emptying the dishwasher—now that's boring! These exercises are challenging, and you will feel a great sense of accomplishment once you have mastered them. Also, you don't have to spend a lot of time doing them each day (see your diary for specifics on time commitment). However, you MUST find the time to do them six days a week. I usually do them after my run, and before I take a shower. Do them on a nice cushy rug or a yoga mat.

THE WORK-OFF STRETCHER

STANDING HIP STRETCH

In a standing position with your legs a little wider than your hips, place your right hand against your right hip. Stretch your left arm up and over your head to the right. Stretch and hold for 5 seconds. Look in the direction you are stretching—brace and push your hand against your hip, and really s-t-r-e-t-c-h that opposite hip and side. Repeat on the other side.

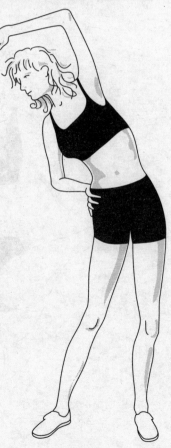

GENTLE INNER THIGH STRETCH

Press gently down on your knees for 15 seconds—keep your back straight.

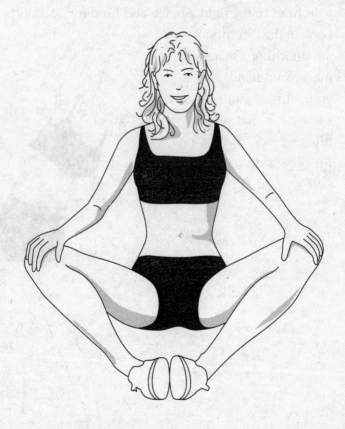

THIGH PULL-BACK

In a seated position with your right leg straight out, comfortably curl your left leg behind you, and hold a gentle stretch. Hold it for 15 seconds, then change legs; remember to keep your back straight.

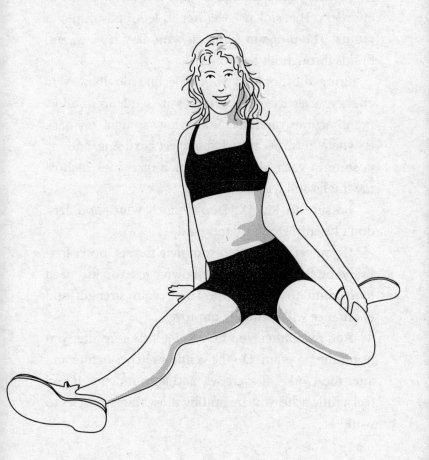

The guiding principle for success is FOCUS. Do each movement slowly, with control. Feel each exercise. Which muscle is tightening and working? Concentrate. Think of yourself as a graceful ballerina with an audience of a thousand or more devoted fans!

At first your movements may not feel smooth or effortless. That's okay—feel free to let out a couple of grunts! The program starts off with easy repeats, and builds throughout the 30 days.

Bring the book to your side and do these very effective exercises and stretches in sequence. Follow the directions carefully. Notice how straight my back is, where my arms are, what my feet are doing, and my posture in each photo—and, of course, look at how my thighs and legs are working.

Be sure to RELAX. Don't hunch your shoulders, don't be stiff. Don't try too hard.

If you get too tired to complete the set, don't fret! Everyone should work at their own pace. You just need to commit to do your best and your strength and endurance will gradually improve.

And remember, you may feel a little sore after you begin the program. Do the gentle stretches before and after the Work-Off exercises, and keep moving. If you feel a little ache, you are putting those thigh muscles to work!

THE WORK-OFF EXERCISER

THIGH RAISE

Illustration 1: Lying facedown, raise your legs—just above your knees—so that your feet are a few inches off the ground.

Illustration 2: Bend your knees, keeping your knees off the ground. Start with 5 seconds, and gradually work up to 15 seconds.

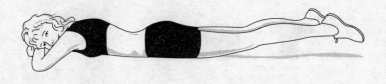

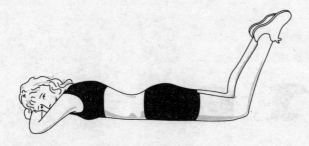

Illustration 1: Slowly unbend your knees.

Illustration 2: Now, with control, lower your straight legs to the ground, then repeat. Begin with 5 reps.

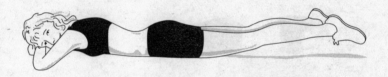

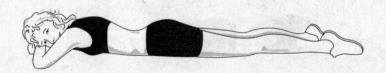

BYE-BYE, INNER THIGHS

Illustration 1: Sit with your back straight, knees bent, and legs wide apart. Place your right arm directly over your right knee, using your left hand to support yourself by your hip.

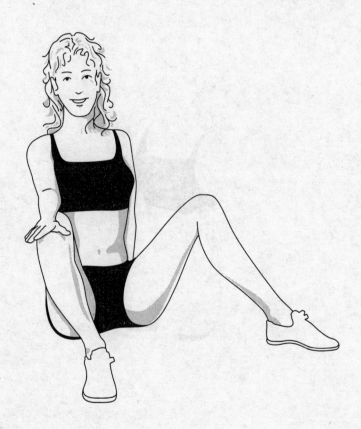

Illustration 2: While sitting straight, touch your left foot to your right hand, and hold for 5 seconds to start. Begin with 5 reps, then repeat on the other side.

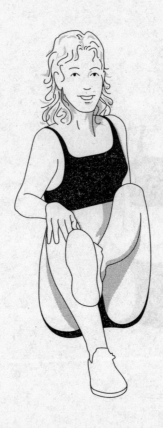

KICK-KICK

Sit as straight as you can, with your right knee bent and left leg straight out. Lift your left leg up so that your foot is at least 6 inches off the ground. Hold for 5 seconds to start, then with control lower the leg. Begin with 5 reps. Repeat on the other side.

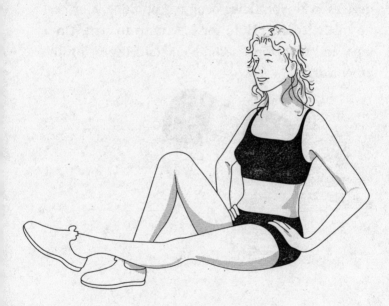

PONY KICK: *Super firming for your thighs and bum.*
Illustration 1: Get down on your hands and knees, with a slight flat incline on your back—do not arch your back in this starting position.

Illustration 2: Slowly raise your left thigh at about 90 degrees, with your knee bent and pointing your heel up to the ceiling. Hold for 5 seconds to start. Do 5 reps, and hold for 5 seconds to start. Repeat on the other side.

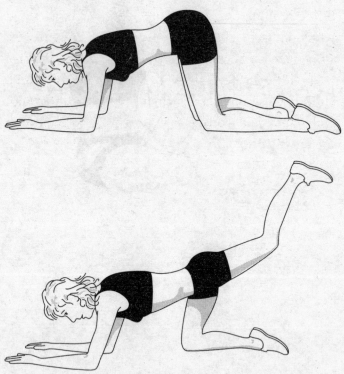

Note: I like to do the following two exercises outside after my Walk-Off, but feel free to do them at home, inside, as part of your Work-Off routine if that is better for you. For these two exercises, I encourage you to access your own fitness level in terms of the number of seconds you hold the pose and the number of reps. Some people progress quite quickly with these, so feel free to push the envelope.

BALLET THIGH

While holding on to a railing or a chair back, stand with both feet facing forward. With your chin up, raise your right leg back at an angle (not straight back)— lead with your heel, about 12 inches off the ground. Hold for 5 seconds, and work up to 10 seconds. Start with 5 reps, and work up to 20 or more reps. Repeat on the other side.

THIGH CHAIR

Illustration 1: Stand about a foot away from a wall (or even a tree) with your feet straight ahead. Slide your body using your arms, until you are sitting with your thighs completely perpendicular to the surface. Don't go down any lower.

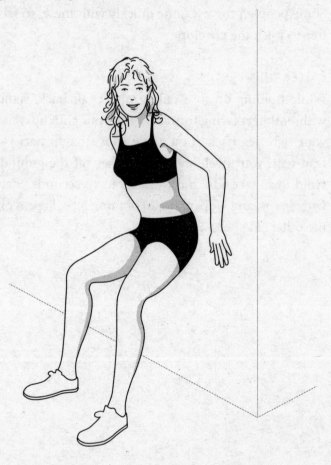

Illustration 2: Hold for 30 seconds to start, and work up until you feel stronger. Do not exceed 2 minutes.

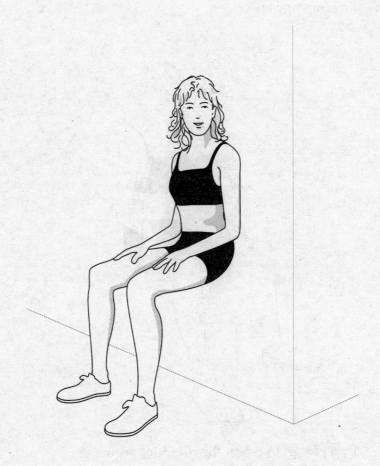

Illustration 3: Spread your thighs wide— hold for 30 seconds, and work up until you get stronger— do not exceed 2 minutes.

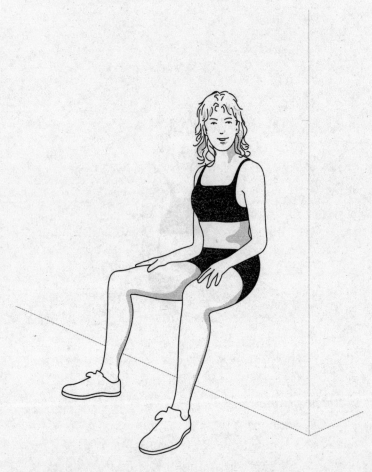

Don't forget to repeat the stretching sequence.

The Walk-Off

||||||||||||||||||||||||||||||||||||||||||||||||||||||||||||||||||||

Walking?! Yes, it's true, this convenient miracle exercise can really slim your thighs. Brisk walking also may reduce the risk of coronary heart disease, stroke, and type-2 diabetes.

Walking BURNS calories. Depending on your pace, you can walk off up to over 300 calories an hour(!), so get your heart pumping, work those lungs, and move those thighs . . . *you will feel great*! You'll steadily create new, tighter, and leaner thigh muscles that will be noticeably firmer.

You'll soon get to love your walk—every day there is something new to see. You can use the Walk-Off for problem solving, dreaming, looking for coins, or counting the flowers. Make it a happy routine!

|||||||||||||||||||||||||||||||||||||||||||||||||||||||||||||||||||

The Thin Thighs in 30 Days Walk-Off program requires walking one to six miles, six days a week depending on your fitness level (see page 18 to determine your fitness level). Also be sure to refer to the Diaries in the back of the book to determine your daily specific goals. The Diaries are a place for you to note your goals and mark off your progress—they help you determine the *minimum* length and intensity required to complete the Thin Thighs in 30 Days Walk-Off program, but (surprise, surprise!) you can always work harder and do more. If you feel ready and would like to, read the Run-Off section that follows on page 56 to learn about how you can incorporate running into your program and burn off even more calories even faster!

BEFORE YOU START YOUR WALK-OFF

- Map out and measure your walking courses. If you are a Beginner, you will need to map out one-, two-, and three-mile courses. If you are Intermediate, you will need to map out two-, three-, four-, five-, and six- mile courses. If you are Advanced, you will need to map out three-, four-, five-, and six-mile courses. Start from your home or use a track (most are ¼ mile around). If you would like to map street or road routes, you can set your car odometer to zero to measure distances. Alternatively, twenty average-size city blocks equal one mile. Where you walk is up to you— you can walk from work and create a lunchtime course or use a treadmill (be sure it can incline). Include hills in your course, or create an optional route with hills.
- Set aside at least 45 minutes (ideally an hour) every day for your Walk-Off (but remember your rest day).
- Get great quality walking/running shoes that leave plenty of room for your toes.

- Do the Work-Off stretching exercises as a warm-up and a wrap-up (they help make your thighs thin).
- Always wear sunblock (at least 30 SPF) when you are outside.
- Choose the Walk-Off level that is right for you.

HOW TO DO THE WALK-OFF

Walk with good posture and your chin held high. Look ahead. Walk naturally (but faster than you typically do), allowing your arms to swing. Remember, you aren't strolling around the mall— step it up several notches! Lengthen your stride to work your inner and outer thighs harder.

Think about what your face looks like when you walk.

Are you frowning or tensing your facial muscles? Relax those muscles. Are your shoulders tight? Roll or shrug your shoulders to loosen them up. Make every step count and really move out to feel your thighs reaching and working to fitness. Smile!

When you first start out, you may feel a little stiff, and the next day you might still feel a little stiff. That may be an indication of some lactic acid buildup and soft tissues that need to be carefully trained up before you add more effort to your routine.

If you become short of breath, slow down; if you become dizzy, stop immediately and regain your equilibrium. You will reap many benefits from walking, even at a slower pace.

Diane met Sam on her daily Walk-Off; a few months later her daily walk-off was a 25-yard jaunt to the altar—and talk about great legs on the honeymoon beach!

READY, SET, WALK-OFF

This program is intense. It is also safe and fun as long as you stay FOCUSED!

Do the warm-up stretches about 10 minutes into your walk. Tendons and muscles need to get slightly warmed up before they are stretched. Study the techniques and know the order in which the stretches are presented so you can remember what you need to do while you are on your walk. And remember, you should repeat this stretching sequence after the Walk-Off.

Warm Up
(IN ORDER)

CALF/ANKLE STRETCH No 1

Stand on a curb or step—get your balance, and learn to do this without support (pretend you have rails under your hands). Bend your right leg slightly, and lower the heel of the left leg. Gently hold the stretch for 10 seconds (do not bounce). Repeat on the other leg.

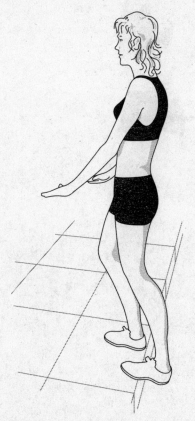

CALF/ANKLE STRETCH No2

Slightly bend your right leg, turning out the left leg at 90 degrees to the side. Turn up your left big toe toward your nose as much as you can. Look at your toe. Hold for 10 seconds. Repeat on the other side.

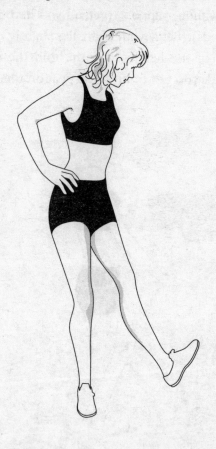

HAMSTRING/INNER THIGH STRETCH

Illustration 1: Find somewhere (at a level that you can manage) to rest your foot on with your leg stretched out. Raise your left leg straight out and reach for your toe— reaching with your nose to your knee. Hold for 10 seconds. Repeat on the other leg.

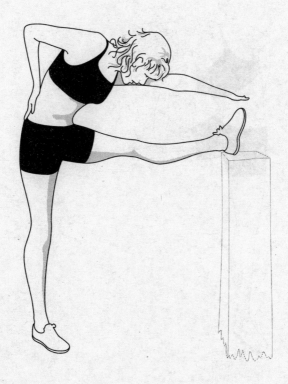

Illustration 2: Stand sideways to your perch, with your back straight, and bring your left elbow to your kneecap. Hold for 10 seconds— really feel a steady stretch. Repeat on the other leg.

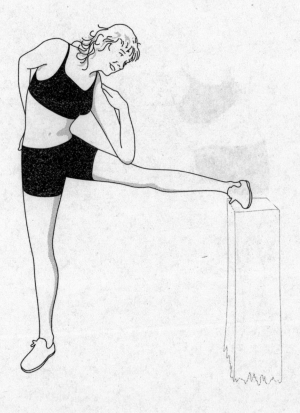

QUAD STRETCH

Stand straight—tuck your bum under you, bend your
right knee, and gently hold your ankle behind you.
Feel the stretch—don't ever try to touch your bum, just
a steady stretch, no strain. Hold for 10 seconds, then
repeat on the other leg.

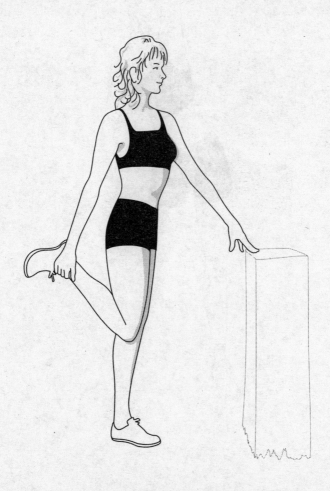

STANDING HIP STRETCH
End with a hip stretch on each side.

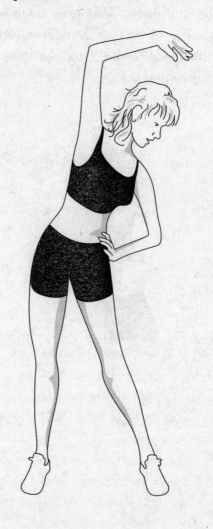

READY, SET, GO!

Once you can walk two miles, you can probably walk four miles. Don't be afraid of distance. After you have your routine established, begin to focus on the "thigh-busting" component. Elite athletes call this part of a workout Interval Training.

BRISK WALK

Keeping chin up, swing your arms freely and cover the ground faster than you typically walk. Get your heart beating.

RACE WALK

Bend your elbows, take faster steps, time yourself. Practice going faster. At intervals, walk as fast as you can!

An interval is a short time period when you change your rate of speed. You should try increasing your speed for an interval. If you are doing brisk walking, mix in short bursts of intense (fast) walking. On my course there is a telephone pole every 200 feet. So I walk (or run) really fast from one pole to the next, and then I go back to my normal speed to the following pole. You can set your intervals to be whatever distance you can manage comfortably.

Here's an example: I typically do about 3 miles of intervals (alternating fast running and power walking), preceded by a ½ mile warm-up, and a walking cool-down. I am in very good shape, so please don't expect that as a goal right now unless you have been walking/running at least 3 times a week for a while.

The trick is to keep the slower interval as short as possible.

Another option is to use time (instead of distance) for marking your intervals. Choose whatever is most convenient and use the diary to guide you. When you do intervals, you will elevate your heart rate, burn more calories, and get thin thighs faster!

Learn to love the hills on your course as they quickly thin those thighs and firm your bum. You also get more of a cardiovascular workout and build strength quicker. After you are comfortable brisk walking on a flat course for at least two miles, add in the hills (start with two). March right up, and then float down. Use your arms as you near the top of the hill to give you that extra push. Try to maintain a consistent speed on your way up.

HILLS:

You will learn to love hills—they make you stronger and work miracles on your thighs. Walk, jog, run looking up ahead, and don't slouch—form counts—

and the hills will be easier. Keep your arms relaxed for the first two thirds of the hill, then put your arms to work—pump them to get you over the crest (an Olympic race trick!).

And here's something more about speed . . . there is a difference between brisk walking and race walking. Brisk will have you a little breathless. It is fast walking with big strides and swinging arms. Race walking is what you might do when you see a sign that reads: "In event of a fire— walk, don't run". Well, pretend there is a fire, and increase the tempo of your strides, increase your arm swing velocity, lean very slightly forward from the waist, and off you go. Race walking is best left for your faster-paced intervals.

TIPS

- Always walk against traffic— never deviate from that rule!
- Don't put yourself in danger by walking/ running alone at night or in unsafe or lonely areas.
- When the temperature is high, be sure to drink plenty of fluids, take it easy, and slow down (especially with temps over 80 degrees).

- Wear really good walking/running shoes—
  they make your walk easier and safer.
- Walk rain (though not thunderstorm) or
  shine and never walk on ice.
- Begin by walking for time (for example, at
  least 30 minutes) and not for distance.

Now off you go on your Walk-Off to a great pair of thighs!

But first, a little bit of inspiration. The following chart notes calories burned and pounds lost for minutes walked:

MINUTES OF WALKING	REDUCTION OF CALORIES	DAYS TO LOSE 5 POUNDS	DAYS TO LOSE 10 POUNDS	DAYS TO LOSE 15 POUNDS	DAYS TO LOSE 20 POUNDS	DAYS TO LOSE 25 POUNDS
30	400	31	62	94	125	157
30	600	23	46	69	92	115
30	800	18	36	54	73	91
30	1,000	15	30	45	60	75
45	400	27	55	82	110	138
45	600	21	42	63	84	105
45	800	17	34	51	68	85
45	1,000	14	28	43	57	71
60	400	25	49	74	93	123
60	600	19	38	58	77	96
60	800	16	31	47	63	79
60	1,000	13	26	40	53	67

After your Walk-Off, be sure to stretch!

THE RUN-OFF

Girls, women, grandmothers— every day I see them outside my front door, running like deer!

Running and jogging are a hundred percent natural for humans. Men and women thousands of years ago spent most of their day either running to catch their food, or running to avoid being eaten. We are built to run.

What are the benefits of running? They are the same as walking. However, running is more difficult cardio work (meaning more calories are burned off and thighs thin faster!). And similar to fast walking, you feel really good after a nice jog or run.

It's easy to begin the Run-Off. When you are doing your Walk-Off, change to a gentle jog for a few minutes, then return to a brisk walk. Do intervals!

If you already run regularly, go to the Advanced program, and you'll do more intervals and more hills.

BEFORE YOU START
1. Have a physical checkup: Are you healthy enough for an intense cardiovascular training program?
2. Have the right shoes. Buy the best brand you can afford. These shoe companies are spending millions on research to make your

run safer and more comfortable. Be sure there is a generous fit—at least a thumbnail from your big toe to the end of the sole. If you look at your street shoes or other leisure shoes, you may see a wear pattern on the soles (for example, more wear on the inside of the shoe sole). Be sure to show that to the shoe salesperson. Shoes should keep your feet balanced and stable. And remember, shoes wear out and you may need at least two pairs each year to keep the stability and cushioning you need.

3. Get a jog bra. Running will not make you sag —in fact, you will actually be using muscles that support your breasts. The jog bra keeps your breasts comfortable and supported.

4. Pick a regular time each day you can devote to your run.

5. Running/jogging can be a wonderful part of your healthy life, so make it a habit. Running is good for your spirits and your health, as well as your thighs!

HOW TO DO THE RUN-OFF

It's important you run/jog with a technique that is natural and comfortable for you. I clomp like an elephant. I don't care—I tried a fancy new stride and got really sore. Be sure you are looking ahead with your chin held high, relax your shoulders, let your arms move naturally, and be sure to watch out for traffic and enjoy yourself! Be aware of pains and aches. You might feel some at first, but keep going. If they don't work out, slow down or stop and resume walking. When you get home, ice the sore area with a bag of ice cubes for about 20 minutes. Never place ice directly on your skin; instead, wrap it with a paper towel. You can also use a bag of frozen peas or a sport ice bag. It is not advisable to stretch the area that hurts. Keep doing your daily program even if your soreness persists, but change back to the Walk-Off. Do warm-up stretches about *10 minutes after* you have done some brisk walking or easy jogging/running (see pages 45 to 50). Your muscles and tendons should be warmed up before you do any stretches.

JOG/RUN

A conversational pace that works for you—don't slouch, and run proud.

FAST JOG/RUN

Pick up your pace—you use this for intervals . . . puff, puff.

BEFORE YOU START

- Choose your level of fitness (see page 18).
- Practise the stretches and do a few in the correct order so you will remember them when you are out on your course.
- Always begin your daily program with walking (even elite runners warm up with walking); don't just run out of the house!
- Treadmill running is effective; you should employ the same techniques as on a course.
- Do intervals—now and then picking up your speed helps make you stronger and gets you in shape to run longer and faster.
- Slow down in the heat—especially when the thermometer is over 80 degrees.
- Always run/jog against traffic—this is a must!

- Running/jogging is a very personal activity —only you can decide when you are ready to run faster or farther. Push yourself at a pace that is now and then challenging and judge when it is time to move to another level. You are in effect your own coach, with the help of this book.
- You are in control of your body—and getting thin thighs is a wonderful result of your dedication!

Off you go for a lovely jog—and don't forget to do your stretches when you're done!

The Weight-Off

||||||||||||||||||||||||||||||||||||||||||||||||||||||||||||||

Congratulations . . . you are now ready to begin your Work-Off and Walk-Off programs, and you're well on your way to firmer and sleeker thighs! Exercise combined with dieting is much more effective than exercise on its own. That's because active muscle cells need more body energy (calories) to keep moving than inactive fat cells do. Muscles burn calories so, even in a resting state, the fitter you are the more calories you'll be burning just sitting on the couch! Take a look at the following chart, and I guarantee you will feel that much more inspired as you work through your Work-Off and Walk-Off programs each day!

ACTIVITY AND CALORIC REQUIREMENTS

WEIGHT	INACTIVE*	MILDLY ACTIVE**	MEDIUM ACTIVE†	ACTIVE‡	VERY ACTIVE§
95	1,140	1,300	1,520	1,710	1,900
98	1,176	1,372	1,568	1,764	1,960
101	1,212	1,414	1,616	1,818	2,020
105	1,260	1,470	1,680	1,890	2,100
110	1,320	1,540	1,760	1,980	2,200
115	1,380	1,615	1,840	2,070	2,300
120	1,440	1,680	1,920	2,160	2,400
125	1,500	1,750	2,000	2,250	2,500
130	1,560	1,820	2,080	2,340	2,600
135	1,620	1,890	2,160	2,430	2,700
140	1,680	1,960	2,240	2,520	2,800
145	1,740	2,030	2,320	2,610	2,900
150	1,800	2,100	2,400	2,700	3,000
155	1,860	2,170	2,480	2,790	3,100
160	1,920	2,240	2,560	2,880	3,200
165	1,980	2,310	2,640	2,970	3,300
175	2,100	2,450	2,800	3,150	3,500
185	2,220	2,590	2,960	3,330	3,700
195	2,340	2,730	3,120	3,510	3,900
200	2,400	2,800	3,200	3,600	4,000
210	2,520	2,940	3,360	3,780	4,200
220	2,640	3,080	3,520	3,960	4,400

* Does nothing actively: Multiply your weight by 12.
** Rides a bicycle to work, sits at work: Multiply your weight by 14.
† Teacher, mother of small children: Multiply your weight by 16.
‡ On the move most of the time: Multiply your weight by 18.
§ Physical worker plus extra exercise: Multiply your weight by 20.

But there's a catch! Exercising more is not an excuse for eating more. Burning more calories than you eat will reduce your body fat . . . but it takes only a small candy bar to ruin the benefits of a lovely Walk-Off!

For most of us, a little dieting is in order to make sure the inches peel off. The Weight-Off is a great program that works!

BEFORE YOU BEGIN

Look in the mirror—are you a size or two larger than you want to be? Do you weigh more than you feel good about? Are you prepared to eat less to keep your new lower weight—not just for few months but for the long term?

Let's talk about motivation. You have to want to be thinner. It is something you must visualize: your body, thinner and healthier. Your desire to lose weight has to be greater than your desire to reach for that fresh baked roll and slather it with butter! We lead our lives around food . . . planning and preparing meals, eating in new restaurants, enjoying a pizza break at work. Often we eat when we aren't even hungry. And, oh boy—the guilt.

To stop eating, you must set a goal, be it a new

dress size, inches off your thighs, or a target weight. For me it was getting inches off my thighs.

Set your sights on being happy, leading a normal life, and eating normal foods. If you are very overweight, find support in a diet program, which can make this complex problem easier to solve through structure and the support of others. Don't be shy about consulting a doctor for advice. Nutrition and weight-loss programs—even available at some workplaces—are accessible to just about everyone.

I am not super-skinny, and I don't diet to become super-skinny. What I want to be is trim and healthy. Determine what your own goal is, making sure to keep in mind that, regardless of your desired weight, you will need to make a firm, no-nonsense decision to control what you eat. Forget about yesterday or tomorrow. What are you putting in your mouth right now?

THE WEIGHT-OFF DIET: HOW TO DIET FOR THIN THIGHS

The Thin Thighs in 30 Days Weight-Off is really simple: calorie counting. Yep, good old calorie counting. Nothing fancy . . . no eating only a single food group, no crash diets or weird recipes. Let me repeat: no crash dieting. Gradual weight loss is healthy and permanent weight loss. According to a 2009 study performed by a team of Harvard researchers led by Frank Sachs, Harvard School of Public Health professor of cardiovascular disease prevention and the senior author of the repeated findings, "Weight loss depends on cutting calories rather than any specific diet. People can lose weight eating the food they like to eat just by eating less". That's right, folks—it's that simple. Cut your calorie intake and you will lose weight!

The deal is that you must burn more calories than you eat while eating enough to meet your nutritional needs. In order to lose weight, you want to use stored caloric energy (fat). Every 3,500 calories you eat and don't burn off turns into a pound of stored fat.

Remember—a calorie is a calorie, whether it is in ice cream or lettuce. Ice cream just has greater caloric density, so if you're counting calories, it's best to determine which foods will actually fill you up and help your body run its smoothest. Maybe skip the ice cream and eat more lettuce?

EAT TO BE WHAT YOU WANT TO BE

The next step? Figure out what your desired weight is and eat only enough calories to achieve and maintain this weight using the chart below. (Remember to be aware of nutrition labels! They're available on almost all food products nowadays, and they'll provide you with all of the information you need to count your calories.)

DAILY MAINTENANCE CALORIES
If you're at your desirable weight

DESIRABLE WEIGHT	18–35 YEARS	35–55 YEARS	55–75 YEARS
99	1,700	1,500	1,300
110	1,850	1,650	1,400
121	2,000	1,750	1,550
128	2,100	1,900	1,600
132	2,150	1,950	1,650
143	2,300	2,050	1,800
154	2,400	2,150	1,850
165	2,550	2,300	1,950

READY, SET, WEIGHT OFF!

In order to design a lower-calorie "daily menu" that works for you, be careful what foods you choose to eat. When I want to drop weight, I go for salads with hard-boiled eggs, veggies with a light drizzle of olive oil, soups, some crunchy whole wheat nutty crackers, shrimp, bananas, baked fish, instant oatmeal, a few almonds or walnuts for a snack, and a multivitamin and mineral supplement so I am sure I am getting all of the vitamins and minerals I need each day. Following are a few tried-and-true tips (believe me, they work!) on getting your calorie intake down so you can lose the weight:

1. Weigh yourself regularly. If it is too stressful for you to do every morning, then choose another schedule. Just do it often and regularly!
2. If you want to eat a cookie, go ahead and treat yourself. Just remember to count it in your daily limit (and don't eat the whole bag like I used to do!).
3. Eat when you are hungry, and never come to the table starving.
4. Watch your salt intake— don't add any to your food.

5. Drink water and stay hydrated. Water can help you feel satisfied and full. Try satisfying hunger with filling "water-foods" like cucumber and melon. Ever see anyone eat a whole watermelon?

7. This is my favorite: Don't eat over the kitchen sink! Sit down and enjoy your food!

8. Pick one food that is calorie-dense that you splurge on regularly (mine was desserts)—and stop eating it.

9. Pick one food that is calorie-dense that you eat at least two times a week (mine was big bowls of pasta with a bucket of Parmesan cheese)—and stop eating it.

10. Pick one 250-calorie food or snack that you eat every day that is calorie-dense (mine was the caramel sauce in my morning latte)—and eliminate it. Stop loading up on those unnecessary calories!

11. Anything else that is calorie-dense that you can safely eliminate? Then eliminate it.

12. Examine the portion size of what you eat and stick to one portion (for example, if you like two pieces of whole wheat toast in the morning, eat just one).

13. Eat with balance—your body needs

calories, fat (less than one-third of your diet fat grams should be saturated fat), carbohydrates, protein, minerals, and vitamins. It does not need refined anything —sugar, bread, and so on. Choose whole grain products, lean meats and poultry, fish, low-fat dairy products, and fresh fruits and vegetables.

14. Check with your doctor before you begin any diet program. Never eat fewer than 1,500 calories a day without being monitored by a physician.

15. Use good sense in budgeting your calories—a roasted chicken breast is 280 calories without the skin and 380 calories with the skin. A cup of sour cream is 496 calories and a cup of plain low-fat yogurt (a delicious substitute) is 144!

16. How many calories do you typically eat in a day? Add them up. Use the food labels with caution. Always look at serving sizes to see how many servings there are in the container—you might be eating four servings and not even know it! And remember, low-fat does not always mean low-calorie! Read those labels to check for the number of calories in each serving.

Look to see what kind of fat is in the food.
Saturated? No, thanks!

For further reading on healthy dieting, I recommend the *American Dietetic Association Complete Food and Nutrition Guide*.

Bon appétit!

CELLULITE: THE FACTS
(AND SOME GOOD NEWS!)

The Big Question: "I have that dimpled fat on my thighs—is that cellulite? And what can I do about it?"

Stephen B. Kurtin, M.D., who has been on the roster of "Top Doctors in America" (Castle Connolly) for eleven consecutive years, says, "What we call cellulite is fat, nothing else. There are no toxins or excess fluids floating among the fat cells."

"The cottage cheese–like appearance is due to the fat pushing on a lattice of connective tissue beneath the skin," says Victor Neel, M.D., a dermatologist at Massachusetts General Hospital in Boston. "This mat of connective tissue breaks down more in some people than in others."

I have not seen any credible clinical research that

indicates that creams, or even liposuction, affect the appearance of cellulite as much as losing weight and maintaining an exercise regimen for your thighs. Most women (including teenagers) have this dimpled fat thing going on.

The good news is that losing weight and developing stronger muscles and firmer thighs can reduce the appearance of cellulite.

Take this test: Sit on a chair in front of a mirror. Cross your legs. Look at the outside of the upper thigh of the leg that is crossed over the other leg. You probably see some dimples on that thigh. Now, really tighten that thigh, make it *look thin*—you will notice that the dimpled fat seems to lessen.

The answer? Lose fat, work to firm those muscles, and get rid of your saddlebags. Your cellulite will also begin to disappear!

THE DIARIES

Diary— Beginner

||||||||||||||||||||||||||||||||||||||||||||||||||||||

Who is a beginner? You are a beginner if you currently do not do a regular cardiovascular program (walking, skating, running, tennis, etc.). By regular, I mean working out three times a week for at least 30 minutes.

Week One

MEASURE YOUR THIGHS, WEIGH YOURSELF

THIGH INCHES: _____ **WEIGHT:** _____

WORK-OFF

Each day (except Monday) do the following:

☐ Begin with warm-up stretches: STANDING
HIP STRETCH, GENTLE INNER THIGH STRETCH,
THIGH PULL-BACK

☐ THIGH RAISE: 5 reps on each leg

☐ BYE-BYE, INNER THIGHS: 5 reps on each leg

☐ PONY KICK: 5 reps on each leg

☐ KICK-KICK: 5 reps on each leg

☐ BALLET THIGH: Remember, for these last
two exercises, go at your own pace. Hold
for 5 to 10 seconds and do 5 to 20 or
more reps.

☐ THIGH CHAIR: Hold for 30 seconds to 2
minutes.

WEIGHT-OFF

Begin to cut calories and establish a daily caloric intake goal. **YOUR DAILY GOAL:** _____

WALK-OFF

SATURDAY: Walk 1.0 mile at a pace faster than a casual stroll. ☐

SUNDAY: Walk 1.5 miles at a pace faster than a casual stroll. ☐

MONDAY: Rest. Focus on your Weight-Off goals and reduce calorie-dense foods from your daily intake. ☐

TUESDAY: Walk 1.0 mile at a brisk pace and introduce intervals into your Walk-Off. For example, walk by three houses at a fast pace and then slow to a brisk pace for the next three houses (walk roughly 30 seconds to 1 minute per interval). ☐

WEDNESDAY: Walk 1.0 mile at a brisk pace. ☐

THURSDAY: Walk 1.0 mile at a brisk pace. ☐

FRIDAY: Walk 1.0 mile at a brisk pace. Find a hill (it doesn't have to be a steep hill, but the longer the uphill slope, the better) and walk up the hill 3 times. ☐

Reminder: Don't forget your stretches during and after your daily Walk-Off!

Week Two

MEASURE YOUR THIGHS, WEIGH YOURSELF

THIGH INCHES: _____ **WEIGHT:** _____

WORK-OFF

Each day (except Monday) do the following:

- [ ] Begin with warm-up stretches: STANDING HIP STRETCH, GENTLE INNER THIGH STRETCH, THIGH PULL-BACK
- [ ] THIGH RAISE: 5 reps on each leg
- [ ] BYE-BYE, INNER THIGHS: 8 reps on each leg
- [ ] PONY KICK: 8 reps on each leg
- [ ] KICK-KICK: 8 reps on each leg
- [ ] BALLET THIGH
- [ ] THIGH CHAIR

WEIGHT-OFF

YOUR DAILY CALORIC INTAKE GOAL: _____

WALK-OFF

SATURDAY: Walk 1.0 mile at a brisk pace.   ☐

SUNDAY: Walk 2.0 miles at a pace faster than a casual stroll.   ☐

MONDAY: Rest. Focus on your Weight-Off goals.   ☐

TUESDAY: Walk 1.5 miles with easy/fast walking intervals. For example, walk by three houses at a fast pace and then slow to an easy pace for three houses (walk roughly 30 seconds to 1 minute per interval).   ☐

WEDNESDAY: Walk 1.5 miles at a brisk pace. ☐

THURSDAY: Walk 1.5 miles at a brisk pace.   ☐

FRIDAY: Walk 1.5 miles at a brisk pace; walk up a hill 5 times.   ☐

Reminder: Don't forget your stretches during and after your daily Walk-Off!

Week Three

MEASURE YOUR THIGHS, WEIGH YOURSELF

THIGH INCHES: _____ **WEIGHT:** _____

WORK-OFF

Each day (except Monday) do the following:

- [ ] Begin with warm-up stretches: STANDING HIP STRETCH, GENTLE INNER THIGH STRETCH, THIGH PULL-BACK
- [ ] THIGH RAISE: 5 reps on each leg
- [ ] BYE-BYE, INNER THIGHS: 10 reps on each leg
- [ ] PONY KICK: 10 reps on each leg
- [ ] KICK-KICK: 10 reps on each leg
- [ ] BALLET THIGH
- [ ] THIGH CHAIR

WEIGHT-OFF

YOUR DAILY CALORIC INTAKE GOAL: _____

WALK-OFF

SATURDAY: Walk 1.5 miles at a brisk pace.   ☐

SUNDAY: Walk 2.5 miles at a pace faster than a casual stroll.   ☐

MONDAY: Rest. Focus on your Weight-Off goals.   ☐

TUESDAY: Walk 2.0 miles with easy/fast walking intervals. For example, walk by four houses at a fast pace and then slow to an easy pace for two houses (remember, walk roughly 1 minute per interval for the fast walking). ☐

WEDNESDAY: Walk 1.5 miles at a brisk pace.☐

THURSDAY: Walk 1.5 miles at a brisk pace.   ☐

FRIDAY: Walk 1.5 miles at a brisk pace; walk up a hill 5 times.   ☐

Reminder: Don't forget your stretches during and after your daily Walk-Off!

Week Four

MEASURE YOUR THIGHS, WEIGH YOURSELF

THIGH INCHES: _____ **WEIGHT:** _____

WORK-OFF

Each day (except Monday) do the following:

- ☐ Begin with warm-up stretches: STANDING HIP STRETCH, GENTLE INNER THIGH STRETCH, THIGH PULL-BACK
- ☐ THIGH RAISE: 8 reps on each leg
- ☐ BYE-BYE, INNER THIGHS: 15 reps on each leg
- ☐ PONY KICK: 15 reps on each leg
- ☐ KICK-KICK: 15 reps on each leg
- ☐ BALLET THIGH
- ☐ THIGH CHAIR

WEIGHT-OFF

YOUR DAILY CALORIC INTAKE GOAL: _____

WALK-OFF

SATURDAY: Walk 2 miles at a brisk pace.   ☐

SUNDAY: Walk 3 miles (or more) at a pace faster than a casual stroll.   ☐

MONDAY: Rest. Focus on your Weight-Off goals and continue to eliminate calorie-dense foods from your diet.   ☐

TUESDAY: Walk 2.5 miles with easy/fast walking intervals. For example, walk by four houses at a fast pace and then slow to an easy pace for two houses (walk roughly 1 minute per interval for the fast walking).   ☐

WEDNESDAY: Walk 2.0 miles at a brisk pace. ☐

THURSDAY: Walk 2.0 miles at a brisk pace.   ☐

FRIDAY: Walk 2.0 miles at a brisk pace; walk up a hill 7 times.   ☐

Reminder: Do your stretches during and after your Walk-Off!

Diary—Intermediate

|||||||||||||||||||||||||||||||||||||||||||||||||||||||||||||||

Who is an intermediate? You are if you walk/run or participate in another cardiovascular program (walking, skating, running, tennis, etc.) at least 3 times a week for 30 minutes or more. You can walk a 13-minute mile. You can walk at least 2 to 3 miles at a brisk pace comfortably.

The plan suggested below can be modified to your own level of fitness. If this program seems light, consider adding miles, intervals, and some short jogs (a minute or two).

Week One

MEASURE YOUR THIGHS, WEIGH YOURSELF

THIGH INCHES: _____   **WEIGHT:** _____

WORK-OFF

Each day (except Monday) do the following:

- ☐ Begin with warm-up stretches: STANDING HIP STRETCH, GENTLE INNER THIGH STRETCH, THIGH PULL-BACK
- ☐ THIGH RAISE: 5 reps on each leg
- ☐ BYE-BYE, INNER THIGHS: 5 reps on each leg
- ☐ PONY KICK: 5 reps on each leg
- ☐ KICK-KICK: 5 reps on each leg
- ☐ BALLET THIGH: Remember, for these last two exercises, go at your own pace. Hold for 5 to 10 seconds and do 5 to 20 or more reps.
- ☐ THIGH CHAIR: Hold for 30 seconds to 2 minutes.

WEIGHT-OFF

YOUR DAILY CALORIC INTAKE GOAL: _____

WALK-OFF

SATURDAY: Walk 3.0 miles at a very brisk pace (hustle and be slightly breathless while walking). ☐

SUNDAY: Walk 4 to 5 miles at a pace faster than a casual stroll. ☐

MONDAY: Rest. Focus on your Weight-Off goals and continue to reduce calorie-dense foods from your diet. ☐

TUESDAY: Walk 3.0 miles with brisk/fast intervals. For example, walk by three houses at a fast pace and then slow to a brisk pace for two houses (walk roughly 30 seconds to 1 minute per interval). ☐

WEDNESDAY: Walk 3.0 miles and push to walk slightly faster than a brisk pace. ☐

THURSDAY: Walk 3.0 miles at a brisk pace (finish with a fast mile—13 minutes or faster). ☐

FRIDAY: Walk 2.0 miles at a brisk pace; find a hill (doesn't have to be a steep hill, but the longer the uphill slope, the better) and walk up the hill 3 times. ☐

Reminder: Don't forget to do your stretches during and after your daily Walk-Off.

Week Two

MEASURE YOUR THIGHS, WEIGH YOURSELF

THIGH INCHES: _____ **WEIGHT:** _____

WORK-OFF

Each day (except Monday) do the following:

- [ ] Begin with warm-up stretches: **STANDING HIP STRETCH, GENTLE INNER THIGH STRETCH, THIGH PULL-BACK**
- [ ] **THIGH RAISE:** 5 reps on each leg
- [ ] **BYE-BYE, INNER THIGHS:** 8 reps on each leg
- [ ] **PONY KICK:** 8 reps on each leg
- [ ] **KICK-KICK:** 8 reps on each leg
- [ ] **BALLET THIGH**
- [ ] **THIGH CHAIR**

WEIGHT-OFF

YOUR DAILY CALORIC INTAKE GOAL: _____

WALK-OFF

SATURDAY: Walk 3.0 miles at a very brisk pace (hustle and be slightly breathless while walking). ☐

SUNDAY: Walk 5.0 miles or more at a pace faster than a casual stroll. ☐

MONDAY: Rest. Focus on your Weight-Off goals.

TUESDAY: Walk 4.0 miles with brisk/fast intervals. For example, walk three houses at a fast pace and then slow to a brisk pace for three houses (roughly 30 seconds to 1 minute per interval). ☐

WEDNESDAY: Walk 3.0 or more miles and push yourself to a faster than brisk pace. ☐

THURSDAY: Walk 3.0 miles at a brisk pace and include one fast (13 minutes or less) mile. ☐

FRIDAY: Walk 4.0 miles at a brisk pace; find a hill and walk up the hill 5 times with momentum! ☐

Reminder: Don't forget to do your stretches during and after your daily Walk-Off.

Week Three

MEASURE YOUR THIGHS, WEIGH YOURSELF

THIGH INCHES: _____ **WEIGHT:** _____

WORK-OFF

Each day (except Monday) do the following:

- ☐ Begin with warm-up stretches: **STANDING HIP STRETCH, GENTLE INNER THIGH STRETCH, THIGH PULL-BACK**
- ☐ **THIGH RAISE:** 5 reps on each leg
- ☐ **BYE-BYE, INNER THIGHS:** 10 reps on each leg
- ☐ **PONY KICK:** 10 reps on each leg
- ☐ **KICK-KICK:** 10 reps on each leg
- ☐ **BALLET THIGH**
- ☐ **THIGH CHAIR**

WEIGHT-OFF

YOUR DAILY CALORIC INTAKE GOAL: _____

WALK-OFF

SATURDAY: Walk 3.0 miles at a brisk pace.

SUNDAY: Walk 4 to 6 miles at a pace faster than a casual stroll. ☐

MONDAY: Rest. Remember your Weight-Off goals! ☐

TUESDAY: Walk 3.0 miles with brisk/fast intervals. For example, walk by four houses at a fast pace and then slow to a brisk pace for two houses (roughly 1 minute per interval for the fast walking). ☐

WEDNESDAY: Walk 4.0 miles and push yourself to a faster than brisk pace. ☐

THURSDAY: Walk 3.0 miles at a brisk pace and include a fast mile (13 minutes or less). ☐

FRIDAY: Walk 3 to 4 miles at a brisk pace; walk up a hill 6 times with momentum! ☐

Reminder: Don't forget to do your stretches during and after your daily Walk-Off.

Week Four

MEASURE YOUR THIGHS, WEIGH YOURSELF

THIGH INCHES: _____ **WEIGHT:** _____

WORK-OFF

Each day (except Monday) do the following:

- ☐ Begin with warm-up stretches: **STANDING HIP STRETCH, GENTLE INNER THIGH STRETCH, THIGH PULL-BACK**
- ☐ **THIGH RAISE:** 10 reps on each leg
- ☐ **BYE-BYE, INNER THIGHS:** 15 plus reps on each leg
- ☐ **PONY KICK:** 15 plus reps on each leg
- ☐ **KICK-KICK:** 10 reps on each leg
- ☐ **BALLET THIGH**
- ☐ **THIGH CHAIR**

WEIGHT-OFF

YOUR DAILY CALORIC INTAKE GOAL: _____

WALK-OFF

SATURDAY: Walk 4.0 miles at a faster than brisk pace.   ☐

SUNDAY: Walk 5.0 miles (or more) at a pace faster than a casual stroll.   ☐

MONDAY: Rest. Don't forget your Weight-Off goals!   ☐

TUESDAY: Walk 3.0 miles with brisk/fast intervals. Use houses or telephone poles to measure your intervals (and remember, do roughly 1 minute per interval for your fast walking).   ☐

WEDNESDAY: Walk 4.0 miles at a brisk pace.

THURSDAY: Walk 3.0 miles at a brisk pace; try to include 2 miles at 13 minutes or faster per mile.   ☐

FRIDAY: Walk 3.0 miles at a brisk pace; walk up a hill 7 times at a brisk pace.   ☐

Reminder: Don't forget to do your stretches during and after your daily Walk-Off.

Diary—Advanced

|||||||||||||||||||||||||||||||||||||||||||||||||||||||||

Who is advanced? You are if you walk/run or participate in another cardiovascular workout at least 5 times each week for 30 minutes or more. You can walk a 12-minute mile. You can walk/run comfortably at least 5 miles at a brisk pace.

The plan suggested below can be modified to your own level of fitness. If this program seems light, consider adding miles, intervals, and more hills and jogging/running (a minute or two at a stretch).

If you are a regular runner, you need to (carefully) increase your mileage and intervals to produce results on your thighs.

Week One

MEASURE YOUR THIGHS, WEIGH YOURSELF

THIGH INCHES: _____ **WEIGHT:** _____

WORK-OFF

Each day (except Monday) do the following:

- ☐ Begin with warm-up stretches: STANDING HIP STRETCH, GENTLE INNER THIGH STRETCH, THIGH PULL-BACK
- ☐ THIGH RAISE: 5 reps on each leg
- ☐ BYE-BYE, INNER THIGHS: 5 reps on each leg
- ☐ PONY KICK: 5 reps on each leg
- ☐ KICK-KICK: 5 reps on each leg
- ☐ BALLET THIGH: Remember, for these last two exercises, go at your own pace. Hold for 5 to 10 seconds and do 5 to 20 or more reps.
- ☐ THIGH CHAIR: Hold for 30 seconds to 2 minutes.

WEIGHT-OFF

YOUR DAILY CALORIC INTAKE GOAL: _____

WALK-OFF/RUN-OFF

SATURDAY: Walk/run 3.0 miles at a very brisk pace (be slightly breathless while walking/running). ☐

SUNDAY: Walk/run 4 to 5 miles at a pace faster than a casual stroll/jog. ☐

MONDAY: Rest. Don't forget your Weight-Off goals! ☐

TUESDAY: Walk/run 4.0 miles at brisk/fast intervals. For example, walk/run by three houses at a fast pace and then reduce to a brisk pace for two houses (roughly 30 seconds to 1 minute per interval) ☐

WEDNESDAY: Walk/run 4.0 miles and push yourself to be faster than a brisk pace. ☐

THURSDAY: Walk/run 4.0 miles at a brisk pace (include 1 fast mile—12 minutes or faster if walking and 9 minutes/mile if running). ☐

FRIDAY: Walk/run 3.0 miles at a brisk pace; find a hill (doesn't have to be a steep hill, but the longer the uphill slope, the better) and walk/run up the hill 5 times with momentum. ☐

Reminder: Don't forget to do your stretches during and after your daily Walk-Off.

Week Two

MEASURE YOUR THIGHS, WEIGH YOURSELF

THIGH INCHES: _____ **WEIGHT:** _____

WORK-OFF

Each day (except Monday) do the following:

- ☐ Begin with warm-up stretches: **STANDING HIP STRETCH, GENTLE INNER THIGH STRETCH, THIGH PULL-BACK**
- ☐ **THIGH RAISE:** 5 reps on each leg
- ☐ **BYE-BYE, INNER THIGHS:** 8 reps on each leg
- ☐ **PONY KICK:** 8 reps on each leg
- ☐ **KICK-KICK:** 8 reps on each leg
- ☐ **BALLET THIGH**
- ☐ **THIGH CHAIR**

WEIGHT-OFF

YOUR DAILY CALORIC INTAKE GOAL: _____

WALK-OFF/RUN-OFF

SATURDAY: Walk/run 4.0 miles at a very brisk pace. ☐

SUNDAY: Walk/run 6.0 miles or more at a pace faster than a casual stroll or jog. ☐

MONDAY: Rest. Remember your Weight-Off goals. ☐

TUESDAY: Walk/run 4.0 miles with easy/fast intervals (roughly 30 seconds to 1 minute per interval). ☐

WEDNESDAY: Walk/run 4.0 or more miles and push yourself to move at a faster than brisk pace. ☐

THURSDAY: Walk/run 3 miles at a brisk pace: include 1 fast mile (12 minutes if walking; if running, 9 minutes or less). ☐

FRIDAY: Walk/run 4.0 miles at a brisk pace and walk up a hill 7 times with momentum! ☐

Reminder: Don't forget to do your stretches during and after your daily Walk-Off.

Week Three

MEASURE YOUR THIGHS, WEIGH YOURSELF

THIGH INCHES: _____ **WEIGHT:** _____

WORK-OFF

Each day (except Monday) do the following:

- ☐ Begin with warm-up stretches: **STANDING HIP STRETCH, GENTLE INNER THIGH STRETCH, THIGH PULL-BACK**
- ☐ **THIGH RAISE:** 5 reps on each leg
- ☐ **BYE-BYE, INNER THIGHS:** 10 reps on each leg
- ☐ **PONY KICK:** 10 reps on each leg
- ☐ **KICK-KICK:** 10 reps on each leg
- ☐ **BALLET THIGH**
- ☐ **THIGH CHAIR**

WEIGHT-OFF

YOUR DAILY CALORIC INTAKE GOAL: _____

WALK-OFF/RUN-OFF

SATURDAY: Walk/run 4.0 miles at a very brisk pace. ☐

SUNDAY: Walk/run 6.0 miles or more at a pace faster than a casual stroll or jog. ☐

MONDAY: Rest. Remember your Weight-Off goals. ☐

TUESDAY: Walk/run 4.0 miles with easy/fast intervals (roughly 30 seconds to 1 minute per interval). ☐

WEDNESDAY: Walk/run 4.0 or more miles and push yourself to move at a faster than brisk pace. ☐

THURSDAY: Walk/run 3 miles at a brisk pace: include 1 fast mile (12 minutes if walking; if running, 9 minutes or less). ☐

FRIDAY: Walk/run 4.0 miles at a brisk pace and walk up a hill 7 times with momentum! ☐

Reminder: Don't forget to do your stretches during and after your daily Walk-Off.

Week Four

MEASURE YOUR THIGHS, WEIGH YOURSELF

THIGH INCHES: _____ **WEIGHT:** _____

WORK-OFF

Each day (except Monday) do the following:

- ☐ Begin with warm-up stretches: STANDING HIP STRETCH, INNER THIGH STRETCH, THIGH PULL-BACK
- ☐ THIGH RAISE: 5 reps on each leg
- ☐ BYE-BYE, INNER THIGHS: 15 reps on each leg
- ☐ PONY KICK: 15 reps on each leg
- ☐ KICK-KICK: 10 reps on each leg
- ☐ BALLET THIGH
- ☐ THIGH CHAIR

WEIGHT-OFF

YOUR DAILY CALORIC INTAKE GOAL: _____

WALK-OFF/RUN-OFF

SATURDAY: Walk/run 4.0 miles at a very brisk pace. ☐

SUNDAY: Walk/run 6.0 miles or more at a pace faster than a casual stroll or jog. ☐

MONDAY: Rest. And always remember your caloric intake goals! ☐

TUESDAY: Walk/run 4.0 miles with brisk/fast intervals (roughly 30 seconds to 1 minute per interval). ☐

WEDNESDAY: Walk/run 4.0 or more miles and push yourself to a faster than brisk pace. ☐

THURSDAY: Walk/run 3.0 miles at a brisk pace and include 1 or more fast miles (12 minutes for walkers and 9 minutes for runners) ☐

FRIDAY: Walk/run 4.0 miles at a brisk pace; walk/run up a hill 7 times with momentum! ☐

Reminder: Don't forget to do your stretches during and after your daily Walk-Off.

Thin Thighs in 30 Days EXPRESS

||||||||||||||||||||||||||||||||||||||||||||||||||||||||||||

With this new and improved version of Thin Thighs in 30 Days, it is now possible to speed up your results—lose inches faster, have firmer, sleeker thighs sooner. Here's how: DOUBLE UP on your daily Thin Thighs in 30 Days program. You can choose how many days a week to do this. Bottom line: When you exercise more often, you become fit faster!

Here is the EXPRESS program:

- Begin your EXPRESS program at a moderate rate for a second daily cardio workout. Walk-Off at about a third of your daily effort for your second daily Walk-Off. So, for example, if you are an intermediate and your daily diary indicates that you should walk 3 miles on your daily Walk-Off, for your second daily Walk-Off walk 1 mile. After two weeks, increase your intensity to where you feel exertion but not soreness. Stay around three-quarters' effort of your first daily Walk-Off for the second Walk-Off of the day.

- Repeat the Work-Off exercises at the same rate but only on the more moderate days (Saturday/Wednesday/Thursday) when the Work-Off is less taxing.
- After your first Walk-Off, drink fluids and eat a light, healthy balanced meal.
- Wait a minimum of five hours before you go back on your course to do your second walk/jog/run and Work-Off.
- Don't eat more calories because of your increased activity!
- The EXPRESS Plan is a great way to start the day and end the day. After 30 days, you'll have even thinner thighs and an even healthier feeling about yourself!

You did it! Now keep up the good work. With regular exercise and by watching your diet, you can maintain your beautifully slim, trim, and sexy new thighs.

WENDY STEHLING, a former advertising and marketing executive, first published her mega-bestseller THIN THIGHS IN 30 DAYS twenty-seven years ago. Today Wendy still follows her programme – and she still has thighs to die for! This classic *New York Times* bestseller has been revised and updated, and is destined to inspire and motivate a whole new generation of women. Wendy lives in Providence, RI.

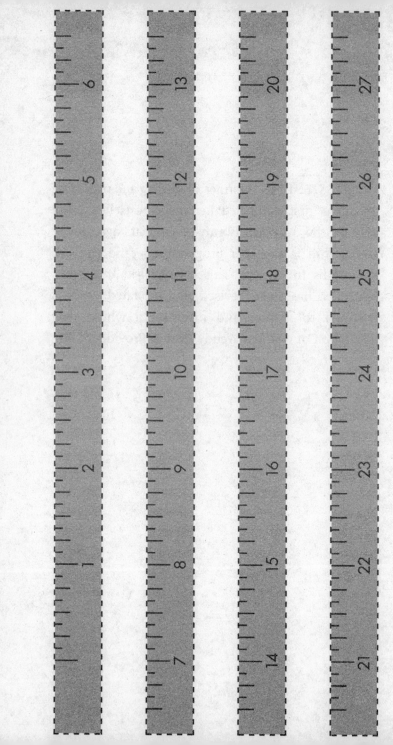

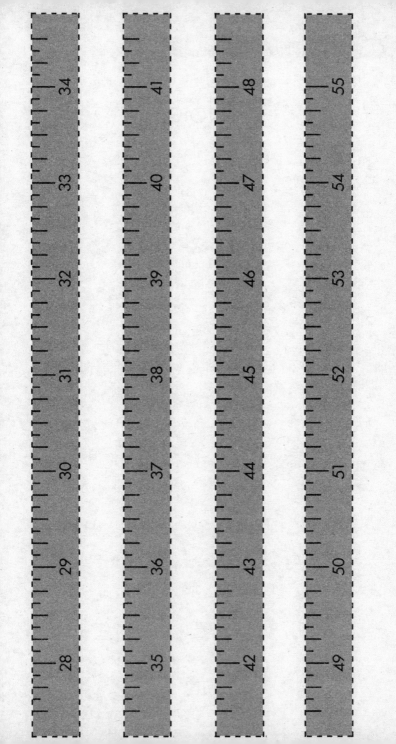

Notes

Notes

Notes